Low-FODMAP
Low-FODMAP
Recipes

Healthy Low-FODMAP Diet Plan &
Recipes Cookbook to Get IBS Relief and
Improve Digestions

The Foods for Healthy Gut

By

WaraWaran Roongruangsri

Simple Book House

Good Health Content

ISBN-13: 978-1530874729
ISBN-10: 1530874726

Part of the secret of success in life is to eat what you like and let the food fight it out inside.

-Mark Twain

CONTENTS

AUTHOR'S NOTE

Attempting to manage your digestive disorder can be tough, particularly if you are in the dark about your illness. For millions of people with IBS, they struggle with everyday tasks, typically when their IBS flares up, however, this is a common illness and nevertheless, so many people do not know how to cope with it.

If you suffer from Irritable Bowel Syndrome, you know that every meal you eat feels like a risk; keeping you on edge as you expect the grief and distress that has ultimately become a very painful part of your daily life.

Thousands of IBS sufferers do not realize just how vital their diet can be, since little changes can actually make a huge difference. If you are eating the wrong food, it will make your condition worse, however by implementing simple changes and slight altering of foods, you can easily learn to manage your IBS.

All you need to do is to figure out what is causing the suffering and you are on your way to finally feeling better—for good—but it can be difficult to find the help you so desperately need.

While IBS and most other digestive disorders are not life threatening, they are not pleasant either, and could lead to serious medical conditions later on in life. Having pain in your stomach is just one issue when your IBS flares up, but by learning how you can deal with it, it can change your life completely.

This book - Low-FODMAP: Low-FODMAP Recipes: Healthy Low-FODMAP Diet Plan & Recipes Cookbook to Get IBS Relief and Improve Digestions, The Foods for Healthy Gut The -Quick Start Guide takes a wide-ranging approach to understanding how you can manage your IBS symptoms through easy dietary deviations, and it provides you with the needed information to help get you started on the Low-FODMAP Diet Plan.

It will provide you with an understanding of just how much high FODMAP foods will affect your body, and will guide you through with what you will need to do in clear and simple steps.

By following all of the guidelines contained in this book, you will bring harmony to your digestion & improve your health and your vitality!

Inside, you will receive:

- Our Low-FODMAP Dieting Approach and Dietary Triggers for your IBS Symptoms
- Our Low-FODMAP Dieting Approach and What exactly are FODMAPs?
- The Effects of FODMAPs on Your Gut
- Our Low-FODMAP Dieting Plan
- Our Guidelines for your Low-FODMAP Dieting Meal Ideas
- In addition - Simple & Delicious & Gut-Friendly Low-FODMAP Dieting Recipes

Thanks for downloading the book! I am sure you will enjoy it!

WaraWaran Roongrungsri

CHAPTER 1:
LOW-FODMAP DIETING APPROACH:
AND DIETARY TRIGGERS FOR
YOUR IBS SYMPTOMS

Introduction

Irritable Bowel Syndrome (IBS) affects almost one in every five Americans. It is a terrible condition that is branded by gut symptoms which include abdominal pains, intestinal gas and wind, bloating, and a change in bowel habits (ranging from diarrhea - constipation). Symptoms can be very debilitating and lead to a reduced quality of life.

A large range of therapies have been used in order to control IBS symptoms, including, but not limited to,

4

various medications, bulking agents & laxatives, and countless lifestyle changes. Almost all people with IBS believe that the symptoms are connected to their ingesting of certain types of foods, nonetheless, advice in this area has always been very conflicting & confusing & offer very little relief for IBS victims.

An Australian research team developed a great dietary approach – Low-FODMAP Diet – used to control symptoms which are associated with IBS.

How to Understand the FODMAP Theory

Carbohydrates (carbs) are present in different forms in your food, fluctuating from long-chain carbohydrates (starch) to simple sugars (glucose) which are digested & absorbed to produce energy. Fiber & resistant starches are long-chain carbs and are resistant to digestion and also important for stool formation & to gain normal bowel function.

The Australian Group has produced solid evidence that a collection of short-chain carbs, named FODMAP's (Fermentable Oligo-saccharides, Di-saccharides, and Mono-saccharides & Polyols) are very problematic for those people with IBS. The short-chain carbs are poorly absorbed into the small intestines and quickly fermented by the bacteria in your gut. The creation of gas by the bacteria is a chief contributor to your symptoms.

An initial study first detected that 3 out of 4 patients who have IBS reacted symptomatically to the restriction of their FODMAP intake. Consequently, several superior clinical studies have further established that improvement was due to reduction in FODMAP intake.

Applications of the FODMAP diet is not only limited to IBS sufferers. It has likewise been shown to improve symptoms in more than 50 percent of the patients with IBS who are experiencing continuing gut symptoms notwithstanding having sedentary disease. In patients who no longer have a colon, the issue of recurrent loose stool production was additionally reduced significantly.

The FODMAP diet can be custom-made to meet your lifestyle and preferences. Following the Low-FODMAP method will not cure IBS, but will allow successful & drug-free management of your symptoms through diet.

CHAPTER 2
LOW-FODMAP DIETING APPROACH: WHAT ARE FODMAPS?

What are FODMAPs?

FODMAP   =   Fermentable   Oligo-Di-Monosaccharides and Polyols

FODMAPs can be found in the foods that we eat. FODMAPs is an acronym for

Fermentable Oligosaccharides: Fructans & Galacto-oligosaccharides (GOS), Fructans which are found in wheat – garlic – onion – inulin, etc. & Galacto-oligosaccharides (GOS) which are found in legumes like beans, lentils, & soybeans, etc.

Disaccharides: lactose which is found in dairy

Monosaccharides: excess Fructose which is found in fruits – honey - & high fructose corn syrup (HFCS), etc.

Polyols: Sorbitol – Mannitol – Maltitol - Xylitol & Isomalt which are found in sweeteners containing isomalt – mannitol – sorbitol – xylitol - & stone fruits like avocado – apricots - cherries – nectarines - peaches - & plums, etc.

FODMAPs are carbs (sugars) that can be found in most foods. There are FODMAPs which are complex names for the collection of molecules found in your food, which can be poorly absorbed by some individuals. When these molecules are poorly absorbed in the small intestines of your digestive tract, the molecules continue along their journey through the digestive tract, arriving at the large intestines, where they will act as a food source to the bacteria that lives there. The bacteria then digests/ferments the FODMAPs and will cause symptoms of Irritable Bowel Syndrome (IBS). Symptoms of IBS include, but are not limited to, abdominal bloating & distension - excess wind (flatulence) - abdominal pain – nausea - changes in bowel habits (diarrhea, constipation - or a combination of both), and other gastro-intestinal symptoms.

Where can FODMAPs be found?

A few instances of food sources for the FODMAPs are listed below. The list is incomplete. New information has been found concerning the FODMAP content of food. Therefore, there have been changes from earlier food lists. Below is a list containing current info. The dietitians at Shepherd Works will better provide you with an up-to-date list of the complete list of food during a meeting.

There are numerous different types of short-chain carbs that make up a FODMAP family. Some of the foods containing these are:

Oligosaccharides: These are comprised of fructans (fructo-oligosaccharides or FOS), which can be made up of short chains of fructose - with a glucose at the end, and galacto-oligosaccharides (GOS), which are short chains of sucrose andgalactose units. These are incapable of being digested, as humans don't have enzymes to break them down. Henceforth, they can't be absorbed in the small intestines and, therefore, will cause problems for patients with Irritable Bowel Syndrome (IBS).

Polyols: They are sugar alcohols, and the most common in the diet are sorbitol & mannitol. Since their absorption is sluggish through the intestinal barrier, only around one-third of what is consumed will actually be absorbed. Therefore, sorbitol is commonly used as a low-calorie sweetener in *sugar free* products, particularly candies & chewing gum.

Excess fructose: Fructose is a very simple sugar & requires no digestion. Although, the absorption of fructose relies heavily on the action of sugar transporters which are located in the wall of your small intestines. Fructose is absorbed in 2 different ways, depending upon how much glucose is present in your foods. First, if glucose is existing in identical or better amounts than fructose, the glucose appears to piggyback the fructose through the small intestinal block. Second, if fructose is in addition to glucose, it will require an alternate absorption technique. This technique of absorption is reduced in some people & is the cause of fructose malabsorption. About 30–40% of healthy & IBS individual's malabsorb additional fructose.

Lactose: Lactose is a disaccharide which is made up of 2 sugar units. It has to be broken down into separate sugar units by an enzyme which is called lactase previous to absorption. Henceforth, lactose is only a FODMAP when there is insufficient levels of lactase - which can be swayed by factors, such as heredities, ethnicity (nearly 100% of Asians and American Indians will have low lactase levels) & many gut disorders.

CHAPTER 3
EFFECTS OF FODMAPS ON OUR GUT

Effects of FODMAPs on our Gut – Fluid Changes & Production of Intestinal Gas

In our small and large intestines, the small FODMAP molecules use an osmotic effect, which means that more fluid is strained into our bowel. FODMAPs are likewise quickly inflamed by colonic microflora-producing gas. This increase in fluid and gas swells our bowel. It will cause the feeling of swelling and abdominal aching or distress, and disturbs how the muscles in the wall of our bowel contract. This may cause amplified advancing movement (peristalsis) which can lead to diarrhea, but in some people, can cause constipation.

It is very important to appreciate that the malabsorption of FODMAPs occurs to a similar extent in well individuals and is a typical phenomenon. It is merely in Irritable Bowel Syndrome (IBS) that gut symptoms are brought more willingly. The reasons for this can include:

a) The means by which the muscles of the bowel reply (motility) to the swelling: They can result in faster or slower passageway through the gut.

b) The gut is "oversensitive" to variations in the gut setting and to relations with the nervous system & immune system in the digestive tract: This means that IBS people are more likely to distinguish pain at a lesser threshold when swelling of the bowel is present, likened to healthy adults.

c) The kind of bacteria in our bowel: The bowel bacteria could yield greater amounts of gas, or there could be amplified bacterial numbers in the small intestines (called small intestinal bacterial overgrowth - or SIBO) so that now more gas is formed in the small bowel. Swelling of the small bowel will cause amplified abdominal uneasiness, distension, & bloating.

CHAPTER 4
THE FODMAP DIET

FODMAPs are osmotic (which means they actually pull water into your intestinal tract), and may not be digested or absorbed very well, and they could be provoked upon by bacteria in your intestinal tract when eaten in surplus.

The symptoms of diarrhea – constipation – gas - bloating and/or cramping will occur in those who are sensitive to the effects of FODMAPs. A FODMAP diet can help to reduce symptoms, which will, in turn, limit foods high in fructose – lactose – fructans - galactans & polyols.

The FODMAP diet is frequently used for people with Irritable Bowel Syndrome (IBS). This diet could be used for those with comparable symptoms ascending from other digestive disorders, like inflammatory bowel diseases.

The diet will limit fiber - because some high fiber foods are high in FODMAPs (Fiber is a constituent of complex carbs which your body can't digest and is found in plant-based foods like beans – fruits – vegetables – and whole grains, etc.)

Food Group	Low-FODMAPs	High FODMAPs (avoid)
Eggs, Meats, Poultry & Fish	Beef – chicken - deli slices – eggs – fish – lamb – pork – shellfish - turkey	made with HFCS/food to limit
Dairy	lactose free dairy (any) - low lactose dairy: cream cheese - half and half - hard cheeses (cheddar – Colby – parmesan – Swiss –	high lactose dairy: buttermilk – chocolate - creamy/cheesy sauces – custard - ice cream - milk (cow, goat, sheep,

	etc.), soft cheeses (brie – feta – mozzarella – etc.), sherbet - yogurt (Greek) - whipped cream	condensed or evaporated), soft cheeses (cottage – ricotta – etc.) - sour cream
Meat, Non-Dairy Alternatives	milk alternatives (almond – coconut – rice - soy (from soy protein) - nuts (walnut – macadamia – peanut – pecan - pine) - nut butters – tempeh – tofu	Cashews – beans - black eyed peas – bulgur – lentils – miso – pistachios – soybeans - soy milk (from soybeans)
Grains	made with gluten free/spelt grains (corn – oats – potato – quinoa – rice – tapioca – etc.): bagels – biscuits – breads – cereals – chips – crackers – noodles – pancakes – pastas — tortillas - waffles oatmeal - oat bran – popcorn – quinoa –	made with wheat/barley/rye when it is the major ingredient - gluten free/spelt grains made with foods to limit - chicory root - inulin

	rice - rice bran	
Fruits	Bananas – blueberries – cantaloupe – cranberries – grapes – honeydew – kiwi – lemon – lime – mandarin – orange - passion fruit – pineapple – raspberries – rhubarb – strawberries - tangerine	Apples – applesauce – apricots – blackberries – boysenberries - canned fruit – dates - dried fruits – figs – guava – mango – nectarines – papaya – peaches – pears – plums – persimmon – prunes - watermelon
Vegetables	alfalfa/bean sprouts - bamboo shoots - bell peppers - bok choy – carrots - cabbage (common) – cucumbers – eggplant - green beans – kale – lettuce – parsnips – pumpkin – potatoes – radishes – rutabaga - seaweed (nori) – spinach – squash – tomatoes – turnips - water chestnuts -	Artichokes – cauliflower – mushrooms - sugar snap peas

	zucchini	
Desserts	made with foods allowed	made with HFCS/foods to limit
Beverages	fruit & vegetable juices/smoothies made with foods allowed (limit to ½ cup at time), coffee - tea	made with HFCS/foods to limit - fortified wines (sherry - port)
Seasonings, Condiments	Jam – jelly - pickle - relish – salsa – sauce - salad dressing made with foods allowed, most spices & herbs - broth (homemade) - butter – chives - cooking oils - garlic/onion infused oil - mustard – mayonnaise - onion (spring green part) – olives – pepper - pesto – salt - seeds (chia – flax - pumpkin - sesame - sunflower) - sugar - vinegar	Chutney – jam – jelly – pickle – relish – salsa - sauce or salad dressing made with HFCS/ foods to limit - agave – garlic - garlic salt/powders – honey – hummus – molasses - onions (brown – leeks – shallots – Spanish – white – spring white part) - onion salt/powders - tomato paste - artificial sweeteners (isomalt – mannitol – sorbitol - xylitol)

Moderate FODMAPs (limit)

There are certain foods that are considered moderate FODMAPs. Follow the serving sizes below for the foods. Avoid these foods only if you have symptoms.

Fruits	Vegetables	Nuts
¼ Avocado	¼ Cup Artichoke Hearts	10 Almonds
3 Cherries	(canned)	10 Hazelnuts
½ Grapefruit (medium)	3 Asparagus Spears	
10 Longon	4 Beet Slices	
5 Lychee	½ Cup Broccoli	
½ Pomegranate (small)	½ Cup Brussels Sprouts	
3 Rambutan	¼ Cup Butternut Pumpkin	
¼ Cup Shredded Coconut	1 Cup Cabbage (savoy)	
10 Dried Banana		

Chips	1 Celery Stick	
	½ Cup Green Peas	
	3 Okra Pods	
	10 Pods Snow Peas	
	½ Corn Cob	
	½ Cup Sweet Potato	

Chapter 5
Guidelines for FODMAP Diet Meal Plan

The presentation of the FODMAP diet necessitates the skilled guidance of a dietician who is trained in the area. A characteristic approach would involve limiting problematic FODMAPs for about **6 to 8 weeks,** or until decent symptomatic control is attained. This will be done by:

- replacing high FODMAP food with lesser options, or
- Decreasing the complete FODMAP capacity consumed at every meal or through the day.

Thereafter, small amounts of FODMAP-containing

food are reintroduced through tasks as advised by the dietician. The goal of this challenge is to slowly increase to levels that are well-tolerated by the individual, while broadening the diet as much as possible. Below is an example menu plan to assist in following the Low-FODMAP diet.

Tips for Low-FODMAP dieting:

Review food list, gather recipes & go grocery shopping initially. When you are ready, begin & follow the diet for six (6) weeks.

- Read all food labels. Avoid food made with high FODMAP fruits and vegetables – HFCS – honey – inulin – wheat – soy - etc. Nevertheless, a certain food could be low in FODMAPs if a high FODMAP food is itemized at the end of the ingredient list.

- Buy gluten-free grains, as they don't have wheat, barley or rye in them. Though, you don't need to be on a gluten-free diet because the emphasis is to limit FODMAPs, not gluten.

- Limit your serving sizes for a low lactose dairy to slight amounts and Low-FODMAP fruits and vegetables to a half cup per meal (½ cup= the size of a tennis ball) if you have signs after eating these foods. The symptoms could be connected to eating big amounts of FODMAPs all at one time.

- Include Low-FODMAP food which are rich in fiber like oatmeal if you develop constipation while on this diet. Drink plenty of water also.

- After the trial period is over, add high FODMAP food one at a time back into the diet in minor amounts so as to identify foods that could be "triggers" to the symptoms. Limit those foods if need be.

Low-FODMAP Meals & Snack Ideas

- Gluten-free waffle with walnuts – blueberries - maple syrup without HFCS

- Eggs scrambled with spinach - bell peppers & cheddar cheese

- Oatmeal topped with sliced bananas, almonds & brown sugar, fruit smoothie mixed with lactose-free vanilla yogurt & strawberries (½ cup)
- Rice pasta with chicken – tomatoes - spinach - topped with pesto sauce
- Chicken salad mixed with chicken – lettuce - bell peppers – cucumbers – tomatoes - balsamic vinegar salad dressing without HFCS
- Turkey wrap with gluten-free tortilla - sliced turkey – lettuce – tomato - slice of cheddar cheese – mayonnaise – mustard, ham and Swiss cheese sandwich on gluten-free bread - with mayonnaise - mustard
- Quesadilla with corn or gluten-free tortilla & cheddar cheese
- Beef & vegetable stew (made with homemade broth – beef - allowed vegetables)

Sample menu selections guide for Low-FODMAP dieting (avoid using elements listed in the <u>high-FODMAP food list</u>)

Breakfast	Gluten-free or spelt toast with spread - sucrose sweetened, *not* with fructose
	Cereal (Oats - Corn Flakes - Rice Krispies)
	Tea or coffee (if you have lactose malabsorption - use lactose-free milk)
	Serving of appropriate fruit
	Poached eggs & spinach
Lunch	Gluten-free or spelt sandwich with fillings (meat – salad - cheese)
	Frittata
	Homemade soup with FODMAP vegetable
	Green salad with dressing (olive oil or lemon juice) and tuna
	Roast pumpkin, goats cheese and

	quinoa salad
Dinner	Meat or fish with Low-FODMAP vegetable or salad
	Baked fish with middle eastern vegetable quinoa
	Roast chicken with rosemary infused vegetables & brown rice
	Gluten-free pizza topped with cherry tomatoes – basil - goats cheese - ham & pineapple
Snacks & sweets	Serving of appropriate fruit
	Yogurt (if you have lactose malabsorption, use lactose-free yogurt)
	Rice cakes with feta
	Gluten-free biscuits
	Berry crumble

CHAPTER 6
SIMPLE AND DELICIOUS GUT-FRIENDLY LOW-FODMAP DIET RECIPES

Main Dish Recipes

Gluten-free Chicken & Vegetable Pie

Ingredients

1 tablespoons sunflower oil

1 garlic of clove, finely chopped

400 g chicken breast fillet, diced

1 med. zucchini, chopped

1 med. carrot, peeled, chopped

1 med. potato, peeled & diced

2 cups gluten-free chicken stock

2 tablespoons gluten-free corn flour

1/4 cup chopped/fresh flat-leaf parsley leaves

1/4 cup fresh tarragon leaves - finely chopped

1 pie pastry (see related recipe)

1 egg - lightly beaten

Directions:

1. Preheat oven to 200°C/180°C fan forced. Heat oil in saucepan over med. heat. Add garlic & chicken. Cook - stirring for 5 minutes or until nicely browned. Add zucchini, carrots and potato. Cook for three minutes. Add one cup of stock to pan.

2. Place corn flour and 1/4 cup remaining stock in bowl. Stir in order to form a paste. Stir in remaining stock. Stir corn flour mixture into chicken mixture. Bring to boil. Reduce heat to medium-low. Simmer for five minutes or until thickened. Stir in parsley & tarragon.

Spoon mixture into a five-cup capacity ovenproof dish.

3. Make pastry: roll pastry out on a lightly floured surface until big enough to cover a dish. Place pastry over filling. Pinch the edges to seal. Brush with egg. Bake for 35-40 minutes or until pastry is golden brown. Let stand for five minutes to cool. Serve.

Nutrition

Energy 1652 kJ

Fat Saturated 3.60 g

Fat Total 20.90 g

Carbohydrate Total 30.80 g

Dietary Fiber 2.30 g

Protein 19.30 g

Cholesterol 75.00 mg

Sodium 622.00 mg

Note

You could use remaining pastry to cut out leaf shapes for decorating the pie top.

Low-FODMAP dieting tip: Make this a FODMAP recipe by leaving out the garlic clove, & replacing sunflower oil with garlic-infused olive oil (available at all delis & gourmet food stores). Also, be sure that chicken stock is onion free.

For recipes classified as gluten free, always check the ingredients to ensure that they do not contain any gluten.

Eggs Florentine

Ingredients

8 thin bacon rashers

20 g. of butter

2 bunches of English spinach, trimmed – washed and dried

Dash white vinegar

4 fresh eggs, room temperature

4 slices ciabatta - sourdough or English muffins - toasted

Hollandaise sauce

1/4 cup (60ml) white wine vinegar

6 black peppercorns

1 shallot - finely chopped

2 egg yolks

200 grams of unsalted butter - melted

2 tablespoons lemon juice

Select ingredients

Directions:

1. Preheat your oven to 200°C/180°C fan forced. Heat the oil in saucepan over

med. heat. Add garlic & chicken. Cook and stir for five minutes or until nicely browned. Add zucchini, carrots and potato. Cook for three minutes. Add one cup stock to pan.

2. Place corn flour and 1/4 cup of residual stock in bowl. Stir to form paste. Stir in residual stock. Stir corn flour mixture in chicken mixture. Bring to boil. Reduce heat to med.-low. Simmer for five minutes or until just thick. Stir in parsley & tarragon. Spoon mixture in a five- cup capacity ovenproof dish.

3. Make pastry: roll pastry out on lightly floured surface until big enough to cover dish. Place pastry over filling. Pinch edges for seal. Brush with egg. Bake for 35-40 minutes or until pastry is golden brown. Let stand for five minutes to cool. And serve.

Nutrition

Energy 3466 kJ

Fat saturated 38.00 g

Fat Total 68.00 g

Carbohydrate sugars 3.00 g

Carbohydrate Total 18.00 g

Dietary Fiber 4.00 g

Protein 37.00 g

Cholesterol 474.00 mg

Sodium 1847.12 mg

Note

Tip: Add vinegar to cooking water when you are poaching eggs and you will immediately set the egg white as it cooks, giving the poached egg an improved shape. Low-FODMAP dieting tip: make this a FODMAP recipe by replacing ciabatta/sourdough/English muffin with toasted gluten-free bread. Omit shallots and use an extra pinch or two of salt in its place.

Mexican Taco Dip

Ingredients:

1 lb. of ground turkey (ground beef can be
used as a cubstitute)

1/2 cup of olive oil

2 14.5 oz. cans of diced tomatoes - drained

1/2 cup of black olives

1 red bell pepper

2 cups of shredded cheese

1/4 cup of cresh cilantro

1/4 cup of fresh chives

1 teaspoons salt

1/2 teaspoon pepper

1/2 teaspoon cumin

1/2 teaspoon paprika

1/2 teaspoon oregano

1/2 teaspoon. dried parsley

1/4 teaspoon cayenne pepper

Directions:

1. Dice red bell pepper in small pieces.

2. On stovetop, grill the ground turkey & diced red bell pepper in olive oil in pan.

3. Add salt – pepper – cumin – paprika – oregano - parsley & cayenne pepper to pan.

4. While grilling, dice cilantro, chives & black olives in small pieces. Set aside.

5. When ground turkey is cooked thoroughly, transfer it, the peppers & spices to medium-sized crock pot, turn on high.

6. Add diced cilantro - diced chives - diced black olives - Diced tomatoes & shredded cheese to the crock pot.

7. Mix thoroughly & cover crock pot.

8. Stir sporadically for the next hour & then turn crock pot to low.

9. Drain excess oil.

10. Serve with tortilla chips, corn tortilla shells and/or taco shells.

11. Continue to stir intermittently throughout the party & after 3-4 hours (or when gone), turn crock pot off.

Note:

> For a spicier mix, add some more Cayenne Pepper or add Diced Jalapenos - Diced Banana Peppers - Diced Green Chilies or Crushed Red Pepper.
>
> Garlic infused olive oil is also great addition due to the fact that it adds the garlic flavor without adding the Fructans.

Roast Broccoli and Salmon

Ingredients:

2 pounds of broccoli

2 tablespoons of extra-virgin olive oil

Salt & pepper (to taste)

4-4 ounce fillets of salmon

1 lemon - cut into wedges

Directions:

1. Preheat your oven to 500F. Cover bottom of large rimmed baking sheet with aluminum foil. Place sheet in oven while oven is heating up.

2. Cut crowns into four wedges. Place broccoli in a large bowl & add olive oil, salt & pepper. Toss to combine. When oven is heated, place broccoli on baking sheet & roast for eight minutes.

3. While broccoli is roasting, prepare salmon fillets by drying them & sprinkling on some salt & pepper.

4. Add salmon on top of broccoli after initial eight minutes of cooking, & roast for an additional eight minutes until salmon is cooked.

5. Remove from oven & squeeze a few lemon slices over top. Serve immediately.

Nutrition

One salmon fillet & ½ pound broccoli is 287 calories - 14.8 g fat - 2.0 g saturated fat - 15.1 g carbohydrates - 3.9 g sugar - 28.4 g protein - 5.9 g fiber - 125 mg sodium - 6 Points+

Rosemary Parmesan Quinoa Polenta Fries

Ingredients:

1 18 ounce tube of Organic Ancient Harvest Quinoa Polenta

2 tablespoons of extra virgin olive oil

½ cup of grated parmesan cheese

⅛ - ¼ cup of chopped fresh rosemary

Directions:

1. Preheat your oven to 425 degrees.

2. Cut polenta tube in half - then cut each half into 16 "fries". You should have 32 fries overall.

3. Place polenta fries on baking sheet lined with parchment paper, & brush olive oil on fries. Place in oven & bake for 45 minutes or until light brown & crispy. You may want to turn the fries every 15 minutes or so to get them extra crispy.

4. When the fries are baking, combine the rosemary & parmesan cheese & set aside in small bowl.

5. Remove fries from the oven when done. Place them on serving dish and sprinkle parmesan cheese/rosemary mixture on top. Serve while nice & hot.

Nutrition: Serving size: 8 fries Calories: 220

Chicken Noodle Soup

Ingredients:

2-3 cup of Chicken Broth

2-3 cups of Water (Fill the Container used for Broth)

1 cup of Cooked, Chopped Chicken Breast

2-4 oz. of Uncooked Gluten-Free Pasta/Noodles (I use Trader Joe's Organic Brown Rice Pasta Fusilli)

Salt and Pepper to Taste

Directions:

1. Add FODMAP Chicken Broth & Water into pot.

2. Bring to boil, stirring frequently.

3. Add Uncooked Gluten-Free Pasta & Chicken to pot.

4. Reduce heat & simmer for around 10 to12 minutes, stirring sporadically.

5. Add Salt and Pepper to taste, if desired.

6. When pasta is cooked to preference, remove from heat.

7. Serve immediately.

8. Makes about four servings.

Note:

The 2 to 4 oz. of Gluten-Free Pasta can be substituted with white/brown rice.

You can refrigerate unused portion & reheat in microwave later.

Potato Soup Recipe

Ingredients:

6-8 large potatoes - peeled and cut in 1 Inch Squares

2 32 oz. containers of chicken broth

1 bunch raw carrots - diced (8 to 10 Large Carrots)

1 bunch green onions - diced (Green Part Only)

1/4 cup of fresh chives, diced

3 tablespoons of garlic in olive oil

2 tablespoons of parsley, diced

3 teaspoons of salt

2 teaspoons of pepper

2 teaspoons of gluten-Free powder

1 teaspoon of dried basil

1 teaspoon of dried oregano

1/2 cup of shredded cheese

1/2 cup of rice milk - warmed

bacon, booked & crumbled as desired (optional)

Directions:

1. Add potatoes – broth – carrots - green Onions & chives into large stock pot.

2. Bring mixture to boil, stirring regularly.

3. Add olive oil – parsley – salt – pepper - powder - basil & Oregano.

4. Reduce heat & simmer for around 30 to 40 minutes or until potatoes are tender, stirring sporadically.

5. Once potatoes have softened, remove from heat.

6. Mash potatoes until well blended.

7. Add Milk & Parmesan Cheese & stir until well blended.

8. Stir in bacon if you are planning to serve immediately. (It isn't recommended that bacon is added prior to freezing.)

9. Garnish with cheese & chives or parsley.

10. Divide into 2 to 3 cup-sized tupperware containers & place in freezer. Makes around 4 to 5 portions.

Note:

Many different items may be added to the soup to make it distinctive or even a bit spicier. Let me know how you make it!

Espresso Crusted Pan Seared Steak

Ingredients:

2 boneless rib eye steaks

1 tablespoon of olive oil, plus a little extra for cooking

2 tablespoons of Espresso (must be espresso **ground**)

1 tablespoon of smoked Paprika

2 tablespoons of chili Powder

1 tablespoon of cumin

1 tablespoon of salt

2 tablespoons of pepper

1 tablespoon of butter

Directions:

1. Rub steaks with olive oil & let come to room temperature.

2. In small bowl combine all spices. Adjust accordingly. (If the little one is not partaking we kick up the heat a bit more)

3. Rub liberally over both sides of steak.

4. Heat cast iron skillet to medium-high & melt butter & a drizzle of olive oil.

5. Cook steaks for 6 minutes each side on medium. Don't poke or lift. 6 minutes. Flip. 6 minutes.

6. Let steaks sit for five minutes before slicing.

Quinoa Tabbouleh with Feta Cheese

Ingredients:

2 cups of water

1 cup of uncooked quinoa

2 teaspoons of sea salt, divided

¼ cup of freshly squeezed lemon juice

2 tablespoons of olive oil

1 cup of thinly sliced green onions

1 cup of chopped fresh mint leaves

1 cup of chopped fresh flat-leaf parsley

5 Persian cucumbers, unpeeled & diced

2 cups of grape or cherry tomatoes, halved lengthwise

1 teaspoon of freshly ground black pepper

1 cup of Feta cheese crumbles

Directions:

1. In a med. sauce pan, bring water to boil. Add quinoa & one teaspoon salt & bring to boil. Reduce heat to low, cover & simmer until water is

absorbed, 15-20 minutes. Transfer quinoa to large bowl & immediately add lemon juice, olive oil & one teaspoon of salt.

2. Gently fold in green onions – mint – parsley – cucumbers - tomatoes & black pepper.

3. Gently fold in Feta cheese & season with additional salt & pepper, if desired. Serve at room temperature or a little chilled.

Mediterranean Baked Fish

Ingredients:

750 g. of baby new potatoes (cut larger potatoes into halves)

250 g. of cherry tomatoes, on the vine

70g of pitted black olives

4 skinless haddock fillets (orsimilar white fish)

2 tablespoons of garlic flavored olive oil

Juice of one lemon

A pinch of salt & pepper

A large handful of fresh basil leaves coarsely chopped or torn

Directions:

1. In a med. sauce pan, bring water to boil. Add quinoa & 1 teaspoon of salt & bring to boil. Reduce heat to low, cover & simmer until water is absorbed, 15-20 minutes. Transfer quinoa to large bowl & immediately

add lemon juice, olive oil & one teaspoon of salt.

2. Gently fold in green onions – mint – parsley – cucumbers - tomatoes & black pepper.

3. Gently fold in Feta cheese & season with additional salt & pepper, if desired. Serve at room temperature or a little chilled.

Dilly Egg Salad

Ingredients:

4 hard-boiled eggs, peeled & chopped

1 tablespoon of mayonnaise

1 tablespoon of spicy mustard

1.5 teaspoons of dried dill

Salt & black pepper, to taste

Directions: Mix all ingredients together.

Greek chicken salad

Ingredients:

2c. of Cubed Cooked Chicken

1 Plum Tomato, small diced

¼ cup of Cucumber, peeled & small diced

12 Pitted Kalamata Olives

½ cup of Crumbled Feta Cheese

½ cup of Hellmann's Mayonnaise

1 tablespoons of Fresh Oregano

2 tablespoons of Lemon Juice

Kosher Salt, if desired

Fresh Ground Black Pepper, if desired

Directions:

1. Pulse chicken in food processor or blender until smooth; place in bowl.

2. Add tomatoes – cucumbers – olives - Feta cheese – mayonnaise - oregano & lemon juice & combine. Season with salt & pepper

Baked Goods Recipes

Chocolate Peanut Butter Bars (no added sugar)

Ingredients

1 cup of dark chocolate chips

1/2 cup of natural peanut butter

2 teaspoons of coconut oil

2 1/2 cup of old fashioned oatmeal

Directions

1. Place sauce pan on stove & heat to med. low heat. Pour in chips, peanut butter & oil. Stirring constantly until melted.

2. Take pan off heat and stir in oatmeal until it is combined with chocolate mixture.

3. Grease 9 X 9 Pan & pour in mixture. Smooth & flatten with spatula.

4. Place in fridge. Let harden for 30 min. to 1 hour. Cut into squares.

5.   Store leftovers in airtight container in
      fridge.

Lemon and White Chocolate Butterfly Cake

Ingredients

Cupcake

> 110 g. (1/3 cup) of softened butter
>
> 110 g. (1/2 cup) of caster sugar
>
> 2 big eggs
>
> 110 g. (1/2 cup) gluten-free self-rising flour
>
> (I use Doves Farm)
>
> ½ teaspoon of baking powder
>
> Grated zest of ½ of a lemon
>
> A few drops vanilla extract

Topping

> 200 g. Lemon curd
>
> 30 g. of white chocolate curls or shavings

Directions

1. Pre-heat oven to 180 degrees C (350F gas 4) & line 12 hole cupcake tin with cases.

2. Place softened butter & caster sugar in large bowl & use electric mixer to cream together until it becomes pale.

3. Add remaining ingredients & continue to mix thoroughly with electric mixer for around a minute until smooth

4. Divide mixture between cases filling them ⅔ full with cake mixture (it makes 9-12 depending on size of your cases)

5. Bake in oven for about 15-20 minutes until golden brown (see if they are ready by placing a skewer in the center, and if it comes out clean, then you know they are cooked through)

6. Cool on wire rack - then cut a circle at the top of each cake & cut the circle in half to make "wings", fill hole with generous teaspoon of lemon curd, sprinkle over white chocolate curls or shavings & place wings on top, pointing upright

Potato Scone

Ingredients

400 g. of floury potatoes, peeled & cut into chunks (I used Maris Piper)

70 g. of self-raising gluten-free flour, with a little extra for dusting (I used Doves Farm)

A good pinch of salt

A little butter or vegetable oil for greasing the frying pan

Directions

1. Place chunks of potato into pan of boiling water & cook until soft (takes about 20 minutes depending on size of the chunks)

2. Mash potatoes and add salt & self-raising gluten-free flour & mix until you have a fairly stiff dough

3. Divide dough into three equal balls - then sprinkle a little gluten-free flour onto work surface & roll balls into circles approximately ½cm thick.

4. Cut each circle into four - then heat frying pan on medium heat & grease with a little butter or vegetable oil

5. Cook in batches of four for 3-4 min. on each side and then cool slightly on wire rack before serving. Great with scrambled eggs.

CHAPTER 7
FINAL THOUGHTS

A varied number of health benefits have been credited to FODMAPs. Fructans – inulin -& GOS are well- known prebiotics, encouraging the growth of valuable bacteria in your gut. For this reason, it is vital to note that **the "Low-FODMAP diet" is *not* a "No FODMAP diet" and it is *not* a "lifetime diet."** I recommend that the diet is followed for at least **6–8 weeks** & then your progress reviewed by a dietician who will aid in advising which foods (and how much) can be slowly re-introduced into the diet.

Breath hydrogen tests can be useful to recognize which partially absorbed sugars – fructose – lactose - & the sugar polyols behave as FODMAPs for each individual. (No breath tests are performed for fructans & GOS [galactooligosaccharides] because they will be malabsorbed in everybody.) For a minority of individuals (less than 2% of community) who don't produce breath hydrogen or methane, breath tests will not provide useful information.

The dietician will ensure that your diet is nutritionally acceptable for you. Many people will return to their usual diet with just a little high FODMAP foods that should be avoided.